Prime Years

The Ultimate Wellness Blueprint for Men Over 50

"Navigating *the Second Half of Life with Health, Happiness, and Purpose*"

J. BOWERS

J. BOWERS

ISBN: 9798870991528

DEDICATION

"Prime Year" is dedicated to those who believe that life is a grand symphony waiting to be composed. To the resilient souls, Purpose driven hearts, The seeker of financial wisdom and the enthusiast of holistic well-being , this book is a tribute to your journey.

CONTENTS

Contents

ACKNOWLEDGMENTS

I extend heartfelt gratitude to all my mentors, contributors and readers.

This composition is a collective effort and your presence adds significant melodies to the narrative.

A special thanks to my editor, thank You for being part of this harmonious journey.

Chapter 1:

Foundations of Physical Health

Chapter 1:

Foundations of Physical Health

Section 1: Understanding the Aging Process

Embracing Change

The journey through the prime years begins with a fundamental understanding of the aging process. Rather than viewing aging as a decline, we approach it as a series of transformations. This section explores the physiological changes that accompany aging and sheds light on how embracing these changes can be a cornerstone of long-term well-being.

1.1 The Dynamic Body

As we age, our bodies undergo a myriad of changes. From shifts in metabolism to alterations in muscle mass, understanding these transformations is pivotal to crafting a tailored approach to physical health. We delve into the science behind these changes, dispelling myths and providing a roadmap for harnessing the body's natural resilience.

1.2 Nutrition Across the Lifespan

Nutrition forms the bedrock of good health at any age, but its importance amplifies in the prime years. This subsection explores the dietary requirements specific to men over 50, emphasizing the role of essential nutrients in supporting overall health. From bone density to cardiovascular health, we unravel the nutritional keys to vitality.

1.3 Exercise as a Lifelong Companion

Physical activity is not just a regimen; it's a lifelong companion. In this section, we navigate the nuances of exercise tailored to the needs of men in their prime years. From strength training to flexibility exercises, we guide you through a holistic fitness approach that aligns with your body's changing dynamics.

Actionable Steps:

Conduct a self-assessment of your current fitness level.

- Explore and incorporate suitable strength and flexibility exercises into your routine.
- Begin to make mindful choices about nutrition, focusing on nutrient-dense foods.

By laying the groundwork for physical health in this opening section, we pave the way for a comprehensive understanding of the body's needs, setting the stage for a fulfilling and active life beyond 50.

Actionable Steps:

1. Conduct a self-assessment of your current fitness level.

Explanation: Before embarking on any wellness journey, it's crucial to have a clear understanding of your current physical condition. Conducting a self-assessment allows you to identify strengths, weaknesses, and areas that may need improvement. This assessment serves as a baseline from which you can track progress and tailor your fitness regimen accordingly.

Examples:

- **Cardiovascular Fitness:** Measure your ability to engage in activities that elevate your heart rate, such as brisk walking or climbing stairs.
- **Strength and Flexibility:** Perform basic exercises like squats, push-ups, and stretches to gauge your current level of strength and flexibility.
- **Mobility:** Assess joint mobility and range of motion through simple movements like shoulder circles, neck rotations, and hip hinges.

2. Explore and incorporate suitable strength and flexibility exercises into your routine.

Explanation: As we age, maintaining and improving strength and flexibility becomes increasingly important for overall well-being. Exploring a variety of exercises and incorporating them into your routine helps address different aspects of fitness, promoting a well-rounded approach to physical health.

Examples:

- **Strength Training:** Include bodyweight exercises (e.g., squats, lunges, push-ups) and resistance training with weights or resistance bands.

- **Flexibility Exercises:** Integrate stretching routines for major muscle groups, focusing on areas prone to tightness, such as the hamstrings, hip flexors, and shoulders.
- **Balance Exercises:** Incorporate activities that enhance balance, like standing on one leg or practicing yoga poses that challenge stability.

3. Begin to make mindful choices about nutrition, focusing on nutrient-dense foods.

Explanation: Nutrition plays a pivotal role in supporting overall health, especially as we age. Making mindful choices about what you eat ensures that your body receives the necessary nutrients for optimal functioning. Emphasizing nutrient-dense foods provides a solid foundation for sustained energy, vitality, and disease prevention.

Examples:

- **Incorporate Colourful Vegetables:** Fill your plate with a variety of colourful vegetables rich in vitamins, minerals, and antioxidants.

- **Prioritize Lean Proteins:** Include lean sources of protein, such as poultry, fish, tofu, or legumes, to support muscle maintenance and repair.
- **Choose Whole Grains:** Opt for whole grains like brown rice, quinoa, and oats for sustained energy and essential nutrients.
- **Stay Hydrated:** Drink an adequate amount of water throughout the day to support hydration, digestion, and overall bodily functions.

By taking these actionable steps, individuals can lay the groundwork for a proactive and personalized approach to their physical health, setting the tone for a vibrant and fulfilling life beyond 50.

Conclusion: Thriving in Your Prime Years

In concluding Chapter 1, "Foundations of Physical Health," we've embarked on a journey to understand and embrace the aging process as a series of transformations, laying the groundwork for a holistic approach to well-being in your prime years. Through the exploration of physiological changes, nutrition essentials, and the importance of tailored exercise, we've set the stage for a proactive and informed approach to physical health.

Reflecting on the Journey

Our exploration began with a shift in perspective – viewing aging not as a decline but as an opportunity for growth and adaptation. By understanding the dynamic nature of the body and the role of nutrition and exercise, we empower ourselves to navigate the prime years with resilience and vitality.

Key Takeaways

1. **Embrace Change:** Acknowledge and embrace the changes your body undergoes, recognizing them as a natural part of the aging process.

2. **Nutrition Foundations:** Cultivate a foundation of good nutrition by understanding the specific dietary needs for men over 50, focusing on a diverse and nutrient-dense diet.

3. **Exercise as a Lifelong Companion:**
Approach exercise as a lifelong companion,
incorporating a variety of activities that
promote strength, flexibility, and overall
fitness.

Next Steps

As you close this chapter, consider the self-assessment of your current fitness level and the incorporation of suitable exercises into your routine. Begin making mindful choices about nutrition, prioritizing nutrient-dense foods that support your well-being.

The journey to thriving in your prime years has just begun. In the chapters to come, we will continue to explore key facets of holistic wellness, including mental resilience, purposeful living, and nurturing relationships. The blueprint for a fulfilling life beyond 50 is unfolding, and you are the architect of your own well-being.

In the words of J Bowers, "Your prime years are an opportunity to not just survive but thrive. It's time to invest in yourself and build the foundation for a life of health, happiness, and purpose."

Turn the page, embrace the journey, and welcome the vitality that awaits you in the chapters ahead.

Chapter 2:

Cultivating Mental Resilience

Chapter 2:

Cultivating Mental Resilience

Embracing the Mind's Landscape

The journey through the prime years is not solely a physical one; it is an exploration of the mind's vast and intricate landscape. In this chapter, we delve into the art of cultivating mental resilience, acknowledging that the mind, much like the body, undergoes its own evolution. As we navigate the complexities of life beyond 50, the ability to adapt, stay mentally agile, and cultivate resilience becomes paramount.

Section 1: Navigating Changes in Cognitive Function

2.1 Embracing Cognitive Evolution

As the years unfold, so does the mind. Cognitive functions, from memory to processing speed, undergo shifts that are both natural and nuanced.

Rather than viewing these changes as obstacles, we explore them as part of a fascinating cognitive evolution. Through engaging narratives and expert insights, we dismantle the stigma surrounding cognitive aging and offer practical strategies to enhance and preserve mental acuity.

Practical Strategies:
- **Mindful Practices:** Integrate mindfulness and meditation into daily routines to enhance focus and cognitive clarity.
- **Brain-Boosting Foods:** Explore a diet rich in omega-3 fatty acids, antioxidants, and vitamins that support brain health.
- **Cognitive Exercises:** Incorporate brain exercises and puzzles that challenge cognitive abilities and promote mental agility.

Section 2: Strategies for Managing Stress and Promoting Mental Well-being

2.2 Navigating Life's Pressures

In the tapestry of life, stress is an inevitable thread. However, how we navigate and respond to stress determines its impact on our mental well-being. This section provides a roadmap for recognizing stressors, implementing effective coping mechanisms, and fostering a resilient mind set in the face of life's pressures.

Practical Strategies:

- **Stress Awareness:** Develop awareness of stress triggers and early signs of heightened stress levels.
- **Mind-Body Connection:** Explore practices such as yoga and tai chi that foster a strong mind-body connection, reducing the impact of stress.
- **Resilience Building:** Learn techniques for resilience-building, including reframing challenges, setting realistic goals, and fostering a positive mind set.

Section 3: Mindfulness and Meditation Practices for Clarity and Focus

2.3 The Power of Presence

In a world filled with constant stimuli, the ability

to be present becomes a superpower. We uncover the transformative effects of mindfulness and meditation, providing not just tools but a philosophy to cultivate a state of presence that enhances mental clarity, focus, and emotional well-being.

Practical Strategies:
- **Daily Mindfulness Rituals:** Integrate short mindfulness practices into your daily routine, such as mindful breathing or a gratitude exercise.
- **Mindful Living:** Embrace the principles of mindful living, bringing awareness to everyday activities for a profound sense of presence.
- **Guided Meditation:** Explore guided meditation practices designed to enhance focus, reduce anxiety, and promote overall mental balance.

The Essence of Mental Resilience

In the tapestry of life, mental resilience is the thread that weaves through every experience. It's not about avoiding challenges but about facing them with a mind that is supple, adaptive, and steadfast. As we immerse ourselves in the cultivation of mental resilience, we recognize that the prime years are an opportunity not just for physical vitality but for a profound and enduring mental flourishing.

In the words of J. Bowers, "The mind, much like a fine wine, matures with depth and complexity. Embrace its nuances, tend to its garden, and watch the flowers of resilience bloom."

Turn the page to embark on a transformative journey into the realms of your own mind. The landscape awaits exploration, and the tools for cultivating mental resilience are at your fingertips.

Section 4: The Wisdom of Emotional Intelligence

2.4 Nurturing Emotional Well-being

In the rich tapestry of mental resilience, emotional intelligence forms an intricate pattern. This section delves into the importance of understanding and nurturing emotional well-being as a cornerstone of mental strength. By exploring the depths of emotions and learning to navigate them with intelligence and empathy, we unlock the door to a more balanced and resilient mind.

Practical Strategies:
- **Emotional Awareness:** Develop a heightened awareness of your emotions, recognizing them as signals for deeper understanding.
- **Effective Communication:** Learn the art of expressing emotions constructively and fostering healthy communication in relationships.
- **Mindful Responses:** Practice responding to challenging situations with mindfulness, allowing for thoughtful and measured reactions.

Section 5: Connecting with Purpose

2.5 Finding Meaning in the Prime Years

As we age, the quest for purpose becomes a guiding light for mental well-being. This section explores the profound impact of finding meaning in life, be it through personal passions, meaningful relationships, or contributing to a greater cause. The intersection of purpose and mental resilience becomes a transformative force, shaping a mind-set that transcends challenges and embraces the richness of experience.

Practical Strategies:
- **Passion Exploration:** Reflect on personal passions and interests, considering how they can be woven into daily life.
- **Relationship Meaning:** Cultivate meaningful connections with family, friends, and the community, recognizing the reciprocal nature of purposeful relationships.
- **Legacy Building:** Explore ways to leave a positive impact, whether through mentorship, philanthropy, or contributing to causes that align with personal values.

The Symphony of Mental Resilience

In the symphony of mental resilience, each instrument plays a crucial role, contributing to the harmony of a well-tuned mind. As we conclude this exploration of cultivating mental resilience, remember that the mind is not static; it is a dynamic and adaptive entity capable of continual growth and transformation.

In the words of J. Bowers, "Mental resilience is not a destination; it's a journey of self-discovery, adaptation, and profound growth. It's the art of turning challenges into stepping stones and finding strength in the symphony of your own mind."

As you turn the page, carry with you the tools and insights to cultivate mental resilience. The prime years are a canvas, and your mind is the paintbrush. Embrace the vibrant strokes of resilience and let the masterpiece of your mental well-being unfold. The journey continues, and the chapters ahead hold the promise of a mind that flourishes with wisdom and resilience.

Conclusion: The Resilient Mind-set

As we conclude this transformative journey through Chapter 2, "Cultivating Mental Resilience," we've navigated the intricate landscape of the mind, exploring its evolution, the impact of stress, and the profound realms of emotional intelligence and purposeful living. In the prime years, mental resilience is not a destination but a dynamic journey, and this chapter has provided the compass to navigate its expansive terrain.

Reflections on Mental Resilience

1. **Adapting to Cognitive Changes:** By embracing cognitive evolution, we dismantle the stigma surrounding aging and open the door to strategies that enhance mental acuity.

2. **Navigating Stress with Grace:** Life's pressures are inevitable, but how we navigate them defines our mental well-

being. Practical strategies empower us to manage stress effectively.

3. **The Power of Mindfulness:** Through mindfulness and meditation, we unlock the transformative power of presence, enhancing mental clarity, focus, and emotional balance.

4. **Embracing Emotional Intelligence:** Nurturing emotional well-being and understanding the depth of our emotions empowers us to build stronger, more resilient minds.

5. **Finding Purpose:** The intersection of purpose and mental resilience becomes a guiding force, shaping a mind-set that transcends challenges and embraces the richness of experience.

Your Resilient Journey

As you embark on the journey to cultivate mental resilience, consider the practical strategies provided in each section. From mindfulness rituals to exploring passions, these tools are not mere concepts but actionable steps toward a resilient mind-set.

In the words of J. Bowers, "Resilience is not the absence of adversity; it's the courage to face it, the wisdom to learn from it, and the strength to grow because of it."

Turn the page with a heart full of resilience, knowing that the chapters ahead hold the promise of a mind that not only endures but thrives. The resilient mind-set is a beacon guiding you through the prime years, illuminating the path to a life rich in wisdom, purpose, and enduring mental strength.

Chapter 3

Purposeful Living in the Second Half

Chapter 3:

Purposeful Living in the Second Half

Unveiling the Tapestry of Purpose

In the symphony of life, purpose is the melody that adds depth, meaning, and resonance. Chapter 3 embarks on a profound exploration of purposeful living, recognizing that the prime years are an opportune time to weave the threads of passion, connection, and contribution into the tapestry of existence.

Section 1: The Significance of Finding Purpose

3.1 Embracing the Essence of Purpose

Purpose is not a distant goal; it is a journey of self-discovery that unfolds in the everyday moments of life. In this section, we delve into the significance of finding purpose, exploring how it shapes our perceptions, choices, and the very fabric of our existence.

Practical Reflections:
- **Clarifying Values:** Reflect on your core values, considering what truly matters to you and aligning these values with daily choices.
- **Defining Personal Mission:** Articulate a personal mission statement that encapsulates your unique purpose, serving as a compass for decisions and actions.

Section 2: Identifying Personal Passions and Interests

3.2 The Journey Inward

Passions are the whispers of the soul, guiding us toward fulfilment and joy. This section encourages a journey inward, exploring personal passions and interests that illuminate the path to purposeful living.

Practical Explorations:
- **Passion Mapping:** Create a visual map of your passions, identifying activities or pursuits that bring joy and a sense of fulfilment.
- **Exploratory Experiences:** Step outside your comfort zone to discover new interests, unearthing hidden passions that may enrich

your life.

Section 3: Setting Goals for Continued Growth and Fulfilment

3.3 The Dance of Aspiration

Goals are the milestones that mark the path to a purposeful life. This section provides a roadmap for setting meaningful and attainable goals, fostering a mind-set of continual growth and fulfilment.

Practical Goal-Setting:
- **S.M.A.R.T. Goals:** Develop Specific, Measurable, Achievable, Relevant, and Time-Bound goals that align with your personal mission.
- **Adaptability:** Embrace the dynamic nature of goals, allowing for adjustments and revisions as you evolve in your purposeful journey.

Section 4: Cultivating Meaningful Connections

3.4 The Tapestry of Relationships

In purposeful living, relationships are the threads

that weave connection, support, and shared meaning. This section explores the vital role of cultivating meaningful connections with family, friends, and the community.

Practical Connection Building:
- **Quality Over Quantity:** Prioritize deep, meaningful connections over a vast network, fostering relationships that contribute to your sense of purpose.

- **Reciprocal Giving:** Recognize the mutual benefits of giving and receiving within relationships, creating a tapestry of support and shared purpose.

Conclusion: Thriving in Purpose

As we conclude this chapter on purposeful living, remember that purpose is not a static destination but a dynamic, evolving journey. Each step taken in the direction of your passions, values, and goals contributes to the creation of a purposeful and fulfilling life.

Key Takeaways:

1. **Purpose as a Guiding Light:** Purpose serves as a guiding light, shaping choices and infusing daily life with meaning.
2. **Passion Exploration:** The exploration of personal passions enriches the journey toward purposeful living.
3. **Goal-Setting for Growth:** Setting goals aligned with your purpose fosters continual growth and fulfilment.
4. **Relationships in Purpose:** Meaningful connections with others contribute significantly to a purposeful and satisfying life.

In the words of J. Bowers, "Purpose is the heartbeat of a fulfilled life. It is the intersection of what brings you joy, what you value, and how you contribute to the world."

Turn the page with a heart attuned to purpose, knowing that the chapters ahead hold the promise of a life rich in meaning, connection, and the ongoing dance of purposeful living.

Chapter 4:

Nurturing Relationships

Chapter 4:
Nurturing Relationships

Unravelling the Threads of Connection

In the grand tapestry of life, relationships form the intricate patterns that define our experiences. Chapter 4 explores the art of nurturing relationships in the second half of life, recognizing the profound impact of meaningful connections on our well-being, happiness, and sense of purpose.

Section 1: Strengthening Connections with Family

4.1 Family Ties: Foundations of Support

Family, the cornerstone of our existence, is a source of strength, love, and enduring connection. This section delves into strategies for strengthening bonds with family members, fostering a supportive network that enriches the journey through the prime years.

Practical Strategies:
- **Open Communication:** Cultivate open and honest communication within the family, fostering understanding and empathy.
- **Shared Rituals:** Establish and maintain shared rituals, whether it's regular family dinners, celebrations, or meaningful traditions.

Section 2: Balancing Personal and Social Life

4.2 The Dance of Social Connection

In the hustle of modern life, balancing personal and social spheres becomes a delicate dance. This section explores the importance of social connection beyond the family unit, highlighting the impact of a rich social life on mental and emotional well-being.

Practical Balancing Acts:

- **Quality Socialization:** Prioritize quality over quantity in social connections, focusing on relationships that bring joy and fulfilment.
- **Boundaries:** Establish healthy boundaries to balance personal time and social engagements, ensuring a harmonious integration of both aspects of life.

Section 3: Building and Maintaining Healthy Partnerships and Friendships

4.3 The Art of Companionship

Partnerships and friendships are the jewels in the crown of a fulfilling life. This section delves into the nuances of building and maintaining healthy, meaningful relationships outside the family circle.

Practical Relationship Building:

- **Communication Skills:** Enhance communication skills to foster understanding and intimacy in partnerships and friendships.
- **Shared Interests:** Cultivate shared interests and activities to deepen connections,

creating a foundation for lasting companionship.

Section 4: Navigating Relationship Challenges

4.4 The Phoenix of Resilient Relationships

Challenges are inevitable in any relationship, but how we navigate them defines the resilience of those connections. This section provides tools and insights for navigating common relationship challenges, fostering growth, and nurturing resilient connections.

Practical Navigation Tools:
- **Empathy:** Cultivate empathy as a guiding force in understanding the perspectives and feelings of others.
- **Conflict Resolution:** Develop effective conflict resolution strategies, emphasizing compromise, active listening, and constructive dialogue.

Conclusion: The Tapestry of Connection

As we conclude this exploration of nurturing relationships, it becomes evident that relationships are not static entities; they are living, breathing threads in the tapestry of our lives. The quality of these threads, whether with family, friends, or partners, profoundly influences our well-being and the richness of our experiences.

Key Takeaways:

1. **Family as Pillars:** Strengthening family bonds provides a solid foundation for support and connection.

2. **Balanced Social Life:** Balancing personal and social life enhances overall well-being, creating a harmonious blend of personal and communal experiences.

3. **Healthy Relationships:** Building and maintaining healthy partnerships and friendships contribute significantly to a fulfilling life.

4. **Resilience in Challenges:** Navigating relationship challenges with empathy and

effective communication fosters resilient connections.

In the words of J. Bowers, "Relationships are the mirror reflecting the essence of who we are. Nurturing them with care and intention creates a tapestry of connection that enriches our journey."

Turn the page with a heart attuned to the intricate dance of relationships, knowing that the chapters ahead hold the promise of a life woven with the threads of meaningful connections.

Chapter 5:

Financial Wisdom for Later Years

Chapter 5:

Financial Wisdom for Later Years

Navigating the Currency of Well-being

In the economic landscape of life, financial wisdom becomes a compass that guides our journey through the later years. Chapter 5 unravels the complexities of financial well-being, recognizing the pivotal role it plays in fostering a secure, stress-free, and fulfilling life beyond 50.

Section 1: Retirement Planning and Financial Security

5.1 Charting the Course for Retirement

Retirement, a new chapter awaiting us, demands strategic planning to ensure financial security and peace of mind. This section explores the intricacies of retirement planning, offering insights into savings, investments, and considerations for a financially stable future.

Practical Planning Strategies:

- **Early Planning:** Emphasize the importance of early retirement planning, understanding the compounding benefits of starting early.
- **Diversified Investments:** Explore diversified investment strategies to mitigate risks and maximize returns, aligning with long-term financial goals.

Section 2: Investment Strategies for Long-term Well-being

5.2 Growing Wealth with Purpose

Investments are the seeds that grow into the trees of financial well-being. This section delves into purposeful investment strategies, considering not just monetary returns but aligning investments with personal values and long-term aspirations.

Practical Investment Approaches:

- **Sustainable Investing:** Consider incorporating sustainable and socially responsible investment practices, aligning financial goals with ethical considerations.
- **Risk Management:** Implement risk management strategies to safeguard investments, acknowledging the dynamic nature of financial markets.

Section 3: Budgeting and Managing Finances

5.3 The Art of Financial Wellness

Budgeting is the brushstroke that paints the canvas of financial wellness. This section provides practical insights into effective budgeting, mindful spending, and managing finances to foster a healthy financial mind-set.

Practical Financial Habits:
- **Budgeting Tools:** Explore various budgeting tools and techniques to track income, expenses, and savings goals.
- **Mindful Spending:** Cultivate mindfulness in spending habits, distinguishing between needs and wants to make informed financial decisions.

Section 4: Ensuring Financial Security in Later Years

5.4 Safeguarding the Future

Life is unpredictable, and safeguarding our financial future involves strategic planning and protective measures. This section explores insurance, estate planning, and other tools to ensure financial security in the later years.

Practical Safeguarding Measures:

- **Comprehensive Insurance:** Evaluate and secure comprehensive insurance coverage, including health, life, and long-term care insurance.
- **Estate Planning:** Develop a thoughtful estate plan, including wills, trusts, and power of attorney documents to protect assets and provide for loved ones.

Conclusion: The Currency of Fulfilment

As we conclude this exploration of financial wisdom, it becomes evident that financial well-being is not just about numbers on a balance sheet; it is the currency that enables a life of fulfilment, choice, and security.

Key Takeaways:

1. **Strategic Retirement Planning:** Early and strategic retirement planning lays the foundation for a secure financial future.
2. **Purposeful Investments:** Aligning investments with personal values contributes to financial well-being with purpose.
3. **Mindful Budgeting:** Cultivating mindful spending habits and effective budgeting promotes a healthy financial mind-set.
4. **Protective Measures:** Safeguarding the future through insurance and estate planning ensures financial security in later years.

In the words of J. Bowers, "Financial wisdom is

not just about wealth accumulation; it's about crafting a life where financial choices align with personal values and aspirations."

Turn the page with a mind attuned to the currency of fulfilment, knowing that the chapters ahead hold the promise of a life where financial well-being becomes a tool for crafting the life you desire.

Section 5: Adapting to Changing Financial Landscapes

5.5 Embracing Financial Flexibility

Life is dynamic, and so is the financial landscape. This section emphasizes the importance of adaptability and flexibility in financial planning. As economic climates change, being open to adjusting strategies and embracing new opportunities ensures continued financial well-being.

Practical Adaptation Techniques:

1. **Regular Financial Check-ins:** Schedule regular assessments of your

financial plan, considering adjustments based on changing goals and external factors.

2. **Continuous Learning:** Stay informed about economic trends, investment options, and financial strategies to make informed decisions in evolving financial environments.

Section 6: Cultivating a Healthy Relationship with Money

5.6 The Psychology of Financial Wellness

Money is not just a tool; it's intertwined with our emotions, beliefs, and values. This section explores the psychology of financial wellness, emphasizing the importance of cultivating a healthy relationship with money for overall well-being.

Practical Mind-set Shifts:
1. **Abundance Mind-set:** Shift from a scarcity mind-set to an abundance mind-set, recognizing opportunities for growth and prosperity.

2. **Financial Education:** Invest in financial education to enhance understanding and confidence in managing money effectively.

Section 7: Planning for Charitable Contributions and Legacy

5.7 Leaving a Lasting Impact

Financial wisdom extends beyond personal well-being; it encompasses the opportunity to leave a positive legacy. This section explores the gratification derived from charitable contributions and the creation of a lasting impact on future generations.

Practical Legacy Planning:
1. **Philanthropic Goals:** Identify causes and organizations aligned with personal values for charitable contributions.
2. **Generational Wealth:** Consider strategies for passing on financial wisdom and resources to contribute positively to the well-being of future generations.

Conclusion: Beyond Numbers, Towards Fulfilment

In concluding this exploration of financial wisdom, it is essential to recognize that the true value of financial well-being extends beyond numerical figures. Financial wisdom is a tool that empowers individuals to craft a life of purpose, choice, and enduring fulfilment.

Key Takeaways:

1. **Adaptability in Finance:** Embrace adaptability in financial planning to navigate changing economic landscapes.
2. **Psychology of Financial Wellness:** Cultivate a healthy relationship with money by understanding the psychological aspects of financial well-being.
3. **Legacy and Impact:** Consider the impact of financial decisions on future generations and explore opportunities for leaving a positive legacy.

In the words of J. Bowers, "Financial wisdom is not just about accumulating wealth; it's about using the power of money to create a life of significance and impact."

Turn the page with a mind-set attuned to the holistic nature of financial well-being, knowing that the chapters ahead hold the promise of a life where financial wisdom becomes a key contributor to a purposeful and fulfilling existence.

Chapter 6:

Holistic Self-Care Practices

Chapter 6:

Holistic Self-Care Practices

Nurturing the Temple: Mind, Body, and Soul

In the intricate dance of life, self-care emerges as the gentle rhythm that sustains the harmony of mind, body, and soul. Chapter 6 explores the profound significance of holistic self-care practices, acknowledging that the prime years are an opportune time to prioritize well-being in its entirety.

Section 1: Integrating Self-Care into Daily Routines

6.1 The Rituals of Self-Care

Self-care is not a luxury; it is a fundamental investment in one's well-being. This section delves into the importance of integrating self-care into daily routines, recognizing that small, consistent practices lay the foundation for enduring health and vitality.

Practical Integration Tips:
- **Morning Rituals:** Establish mindful morning rituals that set a positive tone for the day, incorporating activities such as meditation, stretching, or gratitude practices.
- **Digital Detox:** Integrate periods of digital detox to promote mental clarity and reduce stress, fostering a healthy relationship with technology.

Section 2: Exploring Alternative Therapies for Holistic Well-being

6.2 Beyond Traditional Wellness

Holistic well-being extends beyond conventional practices. This section explores alternative therapies that complement mainstream approaches, offering a holistic perspective on health and self-care.

Practical Exploration Techniques:
  - **Mind-Body Practices:** Engage in mind-

body practices such as yoga, tai chi, or qigong to foster a sense of balance and connection.

- **Holistic Therapies:** Explore alternative therapies like acupuncture, massage, or aromatherapy to address physical and mental well-being.

Section 3: The Role of Sleep, Relaxation, and Leisure

6.3 Recharging the Spirit

In the relentless pace of life, sleep, relaxation, and leisure become essential elements for recharging the spirit. This section emphasizes the profound impact of quality sleep and intentional relaxation on overall well-being.

Practical Restoration Techniques:

- **Sleep Hygiene:** Cultivate healthy sleep hygiene practices, including a consistent sleep schedule, a comfortable sleep environment, and mindful bedtime rituals.

- **Leisure Pursuits:** Engage in leisure activities that bring joy and relaxation, whether it's reading, hobbies, or spending time in nature.

Section 4: Mindful Nutrition for Longevity

6.4 Fuelling the Body, Nourishing the Soul

Nutrition is the cornerstone of holistic well-being, providing sustenance not just for the body but also for the soul. This section explores mindful nutrition practices that contribute to longevity and vitality.

Practical Nutritional Choices:
- **Plant-Based Focus:** Incorporate a plant-based focus in your diet, emphasizing fruits, vegetables, whole grains, and plant-based proteins.
- **Hydration Habits:** Prioritize hydration as a fundamental aspect of nutrition, supporting overall health and vitality.

Conclusion: Thriving in Holistic Well-being

As we conclude this exploration of holistic self-care practices, it becomes evident that well-being is not a compartmentalized concept. It is a tapestry woven from the threads of mindfulness, nourishment, rest, and intentional choices that honour the totality of one's being.

Key Takeaways:

1. **Daily Rituals of Care:** The integration of mindful practices into daily routines forms the foundation for enduring well-being.
2. **Holistic Therapies:** Exploring alternative therapies contributes to a holistic approach to health and self-care.
3. **Spiritual Recharge:** Quality sleep, intentional relaxation, and leisure pursuits are integral to recharging the spirit.

4. **Mindful Nutrition:** Nutrition is a vital component of holistic well-being, fuelling the body and nourishing the soul.

In the words of J. Bowers, "Holistic self-care is not a checklist; it's a dance with the rhythms of life. It is the art of nurturing the mind, honouring the body, and feeding the soul."

Turn the page with a commitment to holistic well-being, knowing that the chapters ahead hold the promise of a life where self-care becomes a celebration of the intricate dance of mind, body, and soul.

Chapter 7:

Embracing Lifelong Learning

Chapter 7:

Embracing Lifelong Learning

The Fountain of Youth: Knowledge and Growth

In the ever-evolving landscape of life, the pursuit of knowledge becomes the elixir that fuels growth, resilience, and a vibrant existence. Chapter 7 explores the transformative power of lifelong learning, recognizing that the prime years are an ideal stage for embracing the joy of intellectual curiosity.

Section 1: The Mind as a Garden of

Possibilities

7.1 Cultivating a Curious Mind-set

Curiosity is the fertile soil in which the seeds of lifelong learning take root. This section delves into the importance of cultivating a curious mind-set, exploring how intellectual curiosity stimulates creativity, problem-solving, and a deep appreciation for the wonders of the world.

Practical Cultivation Strategies:
- **Exploration Challenges:** Engage in exploration challenges that encourage discovering new topics, hobbies, or fields of knowledge.
- **Diverse Reading Habits:** Cultivate diverse reading habits, exploring literature, non-fiction, and genres outside your usual preferences.

Section 2: Embracing Technological Advancements

Navigating the Digital Frontier

In the age of rapid technological advancement, embracing digital tools and platforms becomes essential for lifelong learning. This section explores the opportunities presented by technology, emphasizing how digital literacy enhances access to information, online courses, and collaborative learning.

Practical Digital Integration:
- **Online Courses:** Enrol in online courses to expand knowledge in specific areas of interest, leveraging platforms like Coursera, edX, or Khan Academy.
- **Digital Communities:** Participate in online communities and forums to connect with like-minded learners, fostering collaborative learning experiences.

Section 3: Formal and Informal Learning Pathways

7.3 The Mosaic of Learning Opportunities

Learning is not confined to traditional classrooms; it is a mosaic of formal and informal pathways. This section explores the rich tapestry of learning opportunities, including formal education, workshops, mentorship, and experiential learning.

Practical Learning Exploration:
- **Community Workshops:** Attend workshops and seminars in your community to explore new skills and perspectives.
- **Mentorship Programs:** Seek mentorship opportunities, either as a mentor or mentee, fostering knowledge exchange and personal growth.

Section 4: The Joy of Personal Development

7.4 A Tapestry of Personal Growth

Lifelong learning is not just about acquiring facts; it is a journey of personal development and self-discovery. This section delves into the joy of continuous growth, emphasizing how learning enriches not only the mind but also the soul.

Practical Growth Strategies:
- **Journaling and Reflection:** Incorporate journaling and self-reflection into your routine to deepen the understanding of personal growth.
- **Goal-Setting for Learning:** Set learning goals that align with personal development aspirations, creating a roadmap for continuous improvement.

Conclusion: The Evergreen Spirit

As we conclude this exploration of lifelong learning, it becomes evident that the spirit of curiosity and growth is evergreen. Lifelong learning is not a destination; it is a perpetual journey that invigorates the mind, nurtures the soul, and adds vibrancy to every stage of life.

Key Takeaways:

1. **Curiosity as Catalyst:** Cultivating a curious mind-set is the catalyst for intellectual exploration and lifelong learning.
2. **Digital Literacy:** Embracing technology enhances access to a vast array of learning resources and opportunities.

3. **Diverse Learning Pathways:** Learning is a mosaic of formal education, workshops, mentorship, and experiential pathways.
4. **Personal Growth Journey:** Lifelong learning is a journey of personal development, enriching both the mind and the soul.

In the words of J. Bowers, "Lifelong learning is the dance of the mind with the symphony of knowledge. It is the key to a life that continues to unfold with new possibilities and discoveries."

Turn the page with the spirit of an eternal learner, knowing that the chapters ahead hold the promise of a life where the pursuit of knowledge becomes a source of perpetual joy and fulfilment.

Chapter 8:

Crafting a Legacy of Significance

Chapter 8:

Crafting a Legacy of Significance

Leaving Footprints in the Sands of Time

As we traverse the prime years, the contemplation of legacy beckons—an opportunity to shape the narrative of our impact on the world. Chapter 8 explores the art of crafting a legacy, reminding us that our actions, values, and connections can transcend our own existence, leaving an indelible mark on the sands of time.

Section 1: Defining Legacy Beyond Material Wealth

8.1 Beyond Material Accumulation

Legacy extends beyond material wealth; it encompasses the intangible contributions that resonate with the hearts and minds of others. This section delves into the significance of defining a legacy rooted in values, relationships, and positive influence.

Practical Legacy Definition:

- **Values Reflection:** Reflect on core values that define your character and consider how they can be woven into your legacy.
- **Philanthropic Endeavours:** Engage in philanthropic endeavours aligned with personal values, contributing to causes that make a meaningful impact.

Section 2: Nurturing Relationships as

a Core Legacy

8.2 The Enduring Impact of Connections

Relationships form the tapestry of legacy, weaving a narrative of love, support, and shared experiences. This section emphasizes the enduring impact of nurturing meaningful connections as a core aspect of the legacy we leave behind.

Practical Relationship Building:

- **Quality Time:** Prioritize quality time with loved ones, creating memories and deepening bonds.
- **Generational Wisdom:** Share experiences and impart wisdom to younger generations, contributing to the growth of family legacy.

Section 3: Impact Through Mentorship and Guidance

8.3 Guiding the Next Generation

Mentorship becomes a powerful avenue for crafting a legacy of knowledge and guidance. This section explores the transformative impact of mentoring others, passing on wisdom, and contributing to the growth of individuals and communities.

Practical Mentorship Practices:

- **Open Mentorship:** Offer mentorship to individuals within your field or community, fostering growth and professional development.

- **Knowledge Sharing:** Actively share insights, lessons learned, and practical wisdom to empower others on their journey.

Section 4: Creating Artifacts of Influence

8.4 Expressing Legacy Through Creation

Art, literature, and other creative endeavours become artifacts of influence, shaping the cultural landscape and contributing to the collective legacy of humanity. This section encourages the exploration of creative expressions as a means of leaving a lasting impact.

Practical Creative Pursuits:

- **Artistic Endeavours:** Engage in artistic pursuits, whether it's writing, painting, or music, as a medium for expressing personal and cultural legacies.

- **Educational Contributions:** Contribute to educational resources, writing, or other forms of knowledge dissemination that can endure beyond a lifetime.

Conclusion: The Tapestry of Timeless Impact

As we conclude this exploration of crafting a legacy, we recognize that legacy-building is not a one-time act but a continuous weaving of threads, creating a tapestry of timeless impact. The legacy we leave is not measured in years but in the hearts and minds of those touched by our influence.

Key Takeaways:

1. **Values-Driven Legacy:** Craft a legacy rooted in values, contributing positively to the world beyond material wealth.
2. **Nurturing Relationships:** Prioritize meaningful connections, as relationships form the enduring fabric of legacy.
3. **Mentorship and Guidance:** Contribute to the growth of others through mentorship, passing on wisdom and knowledge.
4. **Creative Expressions:** Explore creative endeavours as artifacts that express and contribute to the cultural legacy.

In the words of J. Bower, "Legacy is the echo of our presence that reverberates through time. It is the gift we offer to future generations—a tapestry woven with threads of love, wisdom, and lasting impact."

Turn the page with the intention to craft a legacy of significance, knowing that the chapters ahead hold the promise of a life where every action, connection, and creation contributes to a narrative that transcends the boundaries of time

Conclusion: Prime Years

As we reach the final notes of this transformative journey through the prime years, the symphony of life echoes with the harmonies of wisdom, resilience, purpose, connection, financial well-being, holistic self-care, continuous learning, and the crafting of a legacy. This book has been a compass, guiding you through the vast landscapes of existence, offering insights, practical strategies, and a tapestry of inspiration to weave into the fabric of your own narrative.

Embracing the Essence of Prime Years

The prime years are not a mere passage of time; they are a canvas waiting for the strokes of intention, passion, and purpose. Each chapter has unveiled a facet of this beautiful canvas, inviting you to embrace the essence of these years as a time of growth, exploration, and profound self-discovery.

Your Journey Continues

As you turn the page and step into the chapters that await, carry with you the echoes of resilience in the face of challenges, the wisdom gained from a life well-lived, and the joy of creating a legacy that transcends the boundaries of time. The prime years are a continuous melody, and your journey is a symphony composed of every choice, every connection, and every moment embraced with intention.

The Author's Hope

In the words of J. Bower, the hope is that this book has served not just as a guide but as a companion on your journey. May the wisdom shared within these pages be a source of inspiration, empowerment, and encouragement as you navigate the landscapes ahead. The symphony of your prime years is uniquely yours, and the crescendo of each day holds the potential for brilliance, purpose, and fulfilment.

A Grateful Farewell

As the final notes of this book fade away, know that the journey continues. Embrace the symphony of your prime years with open arms, knowing that every experience, every challenge, and every triumph contributes to the masterpiece of your life.

In the grand tapestry of existence, your prime years are a symphony waiting to be composed—one filled with melodies of joy, crescendos of growth, and harmonies of lasting impact. May the music of your life be rich, vibrant, and everlasting.

Farewell for now, and may the chapters that lie ahead be filled with the beauty of your unique and extraordinary journey through the prime years.

ABOUT THE AUTHOR

J. Bowers is an experienced, Doctor and Life coach, who brings a wealth of knowledge and practical insights to guide men through the prime years of life. With a focus on evidence-based strategies and a compassionate approach.

J. Bowers empowers readers to make informed choices for a vibrant and fulfilling future.